Alzheimers and You

A Self Help Guide for Sufferers and Carers

Jane E. Hill

authorHOUSE®

AuthorHouse™ UK Ltd.
500 Avebury Boulevard
Central Milton Keynes, MK9 2BE
www.authorhouse.co.uk
Phone: 08001974150

First published by AuthorHouse 1/25/2010

ISBN: 978-1-4490-5371-0 (sc)

This book is printed on acid-free paper.

Index

Introduction

Dr David Somerfield, our mental health consultant, always describes carers as 'the experts.' Only those who have lived with and cared for someone suffering from Alzheimers disease are really able to understand and offer advice on dementia care.

For most of my life I have been a carer, for my father who had Parkinsons Disease, and my husband, Gerald, who has Alzheimers Disease and is also blind. From the start I kept a detailed record of the progress of my husband's illness, how it affected him mentally and physically, and its effect on both of us.

From the onset we both realised that we would have to sell our home in Cheshire which had a large garden. For several years Gerald had gradually lost interest in what used to be his main enjoyment, restoring his beautiful Victorian garden, the garden that he vowed never to leave unless he was carried away 'feet first.'

Four years ago I began my battle to get funding for Continuing Care. I was given invaluable advice from the Alzheimer's Society and Social Services and I have been guided through the system by an army of carers and professionals in the world of mental health. I have learned so much that I feel it is important to pass it on to others who find themselves in a similar situation.

At the end of this book I have included copies of the Decision Support Tools sent me by Torbay Primary Care Trust as well as a complete copy of my presentation to the panel set up by the South West Strategic Health Authority to hear the case. These may provide guidance to anyone who is preparing a presentation. In the first chapter I also provide a short medical history in order to set the scene.

Jane E. Hill

Chapter 1

Early Signs

Aged 49	Heart attack
Aged 59	TIA (Transient Ischaemic Attack),
Aged 77	Hypertension, Macular Degeneration, Glaucoma.
Aged 81	Polymyalgia Rheumatica.
Aged 82	Prostate Cancer, Registered blind.
Aged 83	Diagnosed with Alzheimers Disease.
Aged 85/87	Impaired Kidney Function, Tachycardia, Cellulitis, Urinary Tract Infection, Toxic confusion, Double Incontinence, Total loss of Bodily Control, Shortage of Breath, Chest Pains and Aggression.
Aged 88	Fractured neck of femur

The most common form of Dementia is Alzheimer's Disease, and by 2012 it is likely to affect more than one million of the UK population. At present 20% of our population over the age of 80 suffer from Dementia in one form or another. It is not a normal part of the ageing process. Apart from Alzheimers Disease there are other types of Dementia including Vascular Dementia, Picks Disease and Dementia with Lewy Bodies, whilst other illnesses such as Parkinsons Disease also show similar symptoms.

Dementia is characterised by a progressive decline in mental ability as well as changes in behaviour and personality. There is obvious short term memory loss and also an inability to perform normal everyday activities such as thinking, reasoning, taking decisions and also an inability to concentrate. All the illnesses that are classed as Dementia, are thought to be caused by a combination of factors such as genetics, the environment, diet and general health. Scientists throughout the world are researching the causes and treatment of the disease. In the last few years they have discovered much more about Dementia and are closer to finding a treatment that will prevent or delay the onset of the illness.

Mental and physical deterioration are usually the result of our ability to live longer. We were never meant to live for ever and you may be sure that when dementia and other life threatening illnesses are conquered nature will devise new types of strange or unusual illnesses to bring life to an end.

The heroes and heroines who are responsible for our longevity are the researchers in our universities and medical schools. Whilst politicians dictate what we should eat or the number of glasses of wine we should be allowed to drink, (I wonder how many bottles are consumed in the Dining Room and bars of the House of Commons?)

an increasing number of the population already show early symptoms of Alzheimers Disease and so far no one has yet discovered the cause. Instead of advice from Westminster we need greater funding for Patients, for Carers and for scientific research and patient care. If you have Dementia you need help - and the sooner the better. I have been fighting for help for 10 years.

Are you forgetful ? Really forgetful? Increasingly forgetful? It could possibly be an early symptom of dementia, and if linked to other strange behaviour, such as reversing your car through your closed garage doors - which is what my husband did - it may be even more worrying.

In this book you may read about this odd behaviour and find ways of coping with what is called 'the long goodbye.'

Weeks before his diagnosis other worrying behavioural symptoms showed up. I discovered that Gerald had lost total control of his finances and was happily issuing large cheques to any charity who wrote to him – Cancer Research, Animal Welfare, The RNIB and The Lifeboats, all worthy charities, gained thousands of pounds in a matter of weeks. Whilst I hunted for sufficient money to move house and pay off a bridging loan he visited high quality shops and spent thousand of pounds on expensive furniture.

It soon became obvious that I needed to become involved, or have some control over his financial affairs – luckily the problem was solved by a visit to our solicitor who suggested that it was about time that both of us took out Enduring Powers of Attorney for each other. Fortunately Gerald was enthusiastic about this idea.

Unfortunately he was also enthusiastic about the adverts that came in the post for expensive holidays but when I took a look at his bank statements I discovered that he had already depleted all his reserve savings and had nothing left to draw on for emergencies. Luckily at that stage he was still able to appreciate the seriousness of the situation and together we drew up a savings plan. Looking back I suspect that his blindness, due to Macular Degeneration, was already affecting his ability to read small print and from then on I arranged for his bank and credit card statements to be sent to him in large print. Within weeks our optician had declared him unfit to drive.

Soon Gerald ceased to appreciate the element of danger and risks and in the kitchen he almost caused fires by placing empty pans on the hot plates. On another occasion he went up to the bedroom to change his clothes to go to a party and instead he put on his pyjamas and got into bed. It took me several months to wake up to the fact that there was something wrong somewhere and get him to our G.P. who joined him in his merriment – laughing at my fears – and agreed with him that 'we all get forgetful at times!' After more discussion the G.P. did agree to refer him to a memory clinic which is where the diagnosis of Alzheimer's disease was made. That same year he was also diagnosed with Prostate Cancer and was registered blind.

After several years I learned to recognise the early warning signs of dementia in others, especially when someone relates amusing stories about their friends' odd behaviour, or how their husband used to be a brilliant Bridge player but now cannot remember how to count up his points score.

Early diagnosis enables the patient and their family to plan ahead. Several drugs exist which may affect the rate at which the disease progresses and it is quite usual for patients to try out different medications. At the time of writing the drugs that are available are: Aricept (Donepezil), Exelon (Rivastigmine), Reminyl (Galantamine) and Ebixa (Memantine.) Much has been reported in the national press about the guidance issued by NICE, and the advocacy of the Alzheimers Society who have been successful in their arguments on behalf of patients who were initially refused medication in the early stages of the illness. Thanks to the efforts of the Society many more patients are now able to obtain the medication they so badly need. You can read about these drugs on the fact sheets issued on the Society's web site www.dementiaLink.org/Alzheimers's Society.

When my husband was first diagnosed he was prescribed two drugs that are included in that list, but it soon became clear that they were unsuitable as they caused him to lose his balance. His medication was then changed and he went on to a trial of Ebixa (Memantine). His condition improved noticeably for several weeks, then the improvement halted, but the intensity of the illness also slowed down. Since then he has suffered regular crises in between periods of stability. However I have to accept that these periods of stability may also be influenced by other factors in his daily life such as visits from friends and family at Christmas and Easter. He is now continuing on his trial of Ebixa and I am happy for him to do so. Medication must not raise false hopes and it may take months before a carer or the patient's family are able to detect a change for the better - or for the worse - but changes can, and sometimes do, happen quickly.

When a patient with dementia is on medication it is usual for the consultant to arrange regular appointments for patient check-ups, and nationally recognised memory tests are carried out which give a reliable picture of the progress of the disease. Having attended these regular check-ups with my husband for the last six years I now know all the answers and reckon that I could sail through these questions very easily with the exception of the mental arithmetic tests. I was never much good at mental arithmetic but it seems odd that my husband, who has dementia should achieve higher marks than I could. He may forget people's names, become confused and disorientated and not know where he is, yet he can add, subtract and multiply with only slight hesitation, certainly better than I can.

His clear symptoms began following the onset of Polymyalgia Rheumatica. Until then he had been active in the garden, reading gardening catalogues in the winter and ordering seeds for the coming spring and summer, discussing and planning his planting programme. The pains of Polymyalgia affected his whole body and after only a short time in the garden he had to come into the house to rest. Soon he lost all interest in the garden. He was treated successfully for Polymyalgia with steroids and the consultant was pleased with his progress so that after eighteen months he was declared free of the illness, although it can last much longer for others, however he still complained of pains and was advised to take more exercise. Nevertheless he decided to sell our house and the garden that he had worked in with enthusiasm and dedication for forty years. Despite the regrets of all the family, he decided to move and live in a town near to a Care Village. I believe that at that time he did not expect to live much longer and felt that he might have to be cared for in the nursing home at Nantwich. Although he seemed content to live there I found the area noisy and did not care, at my age, to live so near to a nursing home – I was after all twelve years younger and was not ready to face up to old age. Despite a lengthy search we could not find anywhere else to live in the area and after taking a short break in Devon we decided to move to a beautiful flat in Torquay with a superb view of the sea, overlooking Torbay with views across to Brixham and in the far distance to Weymouth. We have now been living here for eight years. Within weeks of arriving in Torquay my husband was diagnosed with Prostate Cancer, Alzheimers and was registered blind.

Chapter 2

Help!

If like us you live in an area where Social Services, the NHS, and the Mental Health Services all combine to work together and are fully geared up to swing into action and offer you every possible help, then you are lucky. I am told that the same standards do not apply throughout the country.

Social Services, is a vital and important department of your local authority. It is a central cog in the wheel, responsible for assessing all the patient's needs as well as those of the carer. By law it has to carry out detailed assessments of patients and carers. Included in those assessments are the 'sensory' needs for the blind and the deaf and the problems of the very young and the elderly and physically handicapped. Social Services teams are responsible for all the care and assistance that most of us come to rely of at different stages of our lives. They are able to loan equipment for the handicapped and the elderly, and can provide items such as walking aids, supports and adaptations to enable you to get in and out of the bath and move around the house.

In Torbay we have an excellent 'sensory' team that provide visual aids for the blind and deaf and supply useful equipment, such as gadgets that fit onto the rim of your teapot, cup or glass which emit a loud 'beep' when you have poured sufficient liquid into your glass, or hot water into your teapot. If they are really generous they will lend you a large 'easy to see' timing device for the kitchen, a clock that tells you the time when you touch it, and for the deaf there are ear phones that enable you to listen to television programmes, as loud as you like without deafening the rest of the household. They may also be able to supply you with large playing cards so that you can continue to enjoy Whist and Bridge and Poker.

In the South West we have a nationally recognised Low Vision Clinic known as 'Optima,' based at Totnes. The Clinic has an agreement with Torbay Hospital to loan equipment to those who are registered blind or partially sighted. This service is really helpful for the elderly who may sufferer from Macular Degeneration and other eye conditions, and can be tested and fitted with specialist aids and equipped with magnifying glasses.

New equipment is continually being marketed and we found the 'Merlin' reader particularly useful, this enables a patient with poor sight to read a book or newspaper so that the text is deflected and magnified on to a CCTV screen. This is expensive and would obviously be of great use if it were to be installed in the lounge of a residential home – as would large magnifying TV screens and bright angled lamps. In fact help and assistance for the elderly and disabled is probably available quite close to you, but few people ask for help or make use of the opportunities that present themselves. In fact you may be able to apply to your local Rotary Club for a grant to buy aids and services. Unfortunately my husband is no longer able to make use of these excellent machines. He can manage to operate his Talking Book Reader which has been lent to him by the RNIB. By the way the RNIB is always happy to transcribe favourite 'out of print' books on to CD and are grateful for volunteers to help them provide this service.

Computer programs such as 'Word Read' read back text clearly and are simple to use especially for the computer literate.

Anyway back to **Social Services** – Their help and support is never ending. If you have dementia, or are physically handicapped you will be allocated a **Care Manager** whose job it is to monitor your needs and the needs of your carer.

Your Carer? Your Carer is likely to be the most important person in your life and may be a member of your family, a wife or husband, son or daughter or someone appointed by Social Services.

So the team that you will eventually come to rely on is being built up with the help and advice of Social Services.

What about money? Of course all this has to be paid for – one way or another. The dividing line that separates social care from nursing care is obtuse and at the present time, unclear and unsatisfactory. Political arguments continue to rage over funding for what is now known as Continuing Care. As I write this the Government has just issued a new consultation document. In my opinion the options that it puts forward for debate are horrendously expensive, unworkable and have not been costed out and I believe that there many more ways to fund care for the elderly and disabled.

In the following chapter I have attempted to clarify the system which deals specifically with your needs and who pays for them.

You will find that the patient's needs change quite regularly and that you need to make use of all the different types of help that are available. Eventually the time will come when the illness progresses so much that it will become difficult for you to care at home without asking for much more help.

Devon is a retirement area and has an abundant supply of care organisations. Social Services supply information on Home Care organisations, Home Nursing, Carers and Care Homes and will always advise on costs and offer help and advice.

Day Care is also arranged by Social Services. Day Care not only gives the carer time to themselves but should also provide the patient with some mental stimulus. There is no truer saying than 'Use it or Lose it' and if you are blind and receive no mental stimulus your memory deteriorates even more quickly.

Car transport to and from Day Care Centres is usually provided between 10am and 4pm. During the day there are quizzes, singing, discussions, and lunch is provided. It is well known that music and singing does help to improve well being in dementia patients. In some centres patients can also be bathed. Day care is a very useful service and is often provided by Care Homes, especially for those patients who may eventually need to go into a home permanently, also it gives the family of the patient the opportunity to assess whether the home is suitable and the patient is happy there.

Age Concern also provide **Host Carers** who arrange day care in their own homes, taking and collecting older people, providing lunch and in good weather taking the clients out for coffee, lunch or shopping. They try to organise groups of people who share similar interests and get on well together such as ex-service men, Rotarians etc.

Another alternative is **Home care.** Carers are provided in the home by Home Care Organisations who carry out whatever help is needed, dressing, bathing, shopping, cooking etc. They charge by the hour at rates set by Social Services unless there is a private arrangement in place.

In fact all these services can be arranged on a contract by Social Services through the Care Manager and are usually much cheaper than private arrangements.

Respite Care can also be organised by Social Services. This is an arrangement where the patient goes into care for one or two weeks so that the carer can take a holiday. Make no mistake about it carers do need holidays! In some cases where the patient qualifies the carer may be supplied with vouchers which help to pay for their own breaks.

It must be recognised that when a patient goes into a Care Home there is a team of carers, cooks and cleaners, and laundry staff – whilst in the patient's home there is a team of one who carries out all these duties and who needs regular breaks.

During this time I took several short breaks but whenever I returned the problems were still there waiting for me.

When my husband was diagnosed with Alzheimers I thought I would be able to cope with the situation, but after two years I really needed much more help. Continual arguments, aggression and incontinence reduced me to tears of desperation. Social Services suggested that Gerald should go to a Host carer one day a week. This worked well, I enjoyed my day off and he enjoyed the company of the other members of the group so I increased his attendance to two days a week. It may sound as if I was having fun whilst he was away from home, but it did not really work like that for I had to take on all the responsibilities that he had previously dealt with – bills to pay, bank statements to check, correspondence, and forms to fill in as well as taking on an Enduring Power of Attorney and sending copies of the documents to all and sundry as I could not deal with his affairs without proper notification of the situation – and it takes up hours of time.

As he was blind he could not see or drive a car so I became 'chief cook and bottle-washer,' chauffeur and secretary – in charge of and responsible for everything. Of course at the end of the financial year I also had to provide all receipts, dividend counterfoils, bank statements and complete his tax returns. On his days at home I took him to dental appointments, doctor's appointments and visits to opticians as well as getting his hair cut (and the dog to the vets!)

My husband was unable to take a bath without help and as I could not lift him I asked for help from Home care who came twice a week in the mornings to bathe him.

As his condition steadily deteriorated the work increased and I felt the need to have more time off, so we increased his Day Care visits twice weekly to the home where he may eventually have to stay permanently. That means that he is now cared for four days a week. Then I found that he could be bathed when he went to Day Care, so I sent a set of clean clothes with him and they return his soiled clothes to me to wash.

All this sounds a good arrangement, but in fact Care Homes often do mix up patient's clothes, then they return home with some other man's underpants and socks and sometimes they even lose shirts! Obviously it is not satisfactory to be wearing someone else clothes. I am baffled at the inability of Care Homes to come up with a well thought out arrangement to avoid this situation - and put all the soiled clothes back into the same bag! It's not 'Rocket Science!' Anyway after several weeks we eventually worked out a system, although it still breaks down from time to time.

Much trouble, aggression and anger shows up later in the day. Apparently this is quite usual. I am sure that my husband never wanted me to carry out his personal care. He found it embarrassing and it was easier for him to have a professional carer to change his continence pad. If I carried out his evening care he became very difficult, refusing to co-operate, shouting and even throwing his dirty pad at me. So I solved this by arranging for an evening carer to come in and get him ready for bed.

As soon as I managed to solve one problem another one appeared and before long I became totally exhausted and very emotional. I attend church regularly, but at that time I became so overwrought that as soon as the hymn singing began I started to weep and that usually continued throughout the service.

At home I swore and became impossibly intolerant. After 50 years of wonderfully happy marriage and having just celebrated our Golden Wedding it came as a terrible shock to have to cope with his aggression and uncontrollable behaviour. I fell asleep at every opportunity and I also fell over regularly, breaking my hand, tearing a ligament in my leg and spraining my ankle. After only a few months I lost control of my car and crashed it in a motorway car park. I had reached crisis point and I was desperate for help. At last the Doctor prescribed Citalopram, an antidepressant, and after only a few weeks life soon became almost worth living.

Falling

Gerald was described in his hospital report as 'a frail elderly man, at high risk of falling' Eventually in April he fell at home and broke his hip. He was operated on at Torbay hospital and had a total hip replacement and was then moved to Paignton hospital for convalescence. The operation was very successful but unfortunately he quickly lost confidence in being able to walk and despite my insistence the physiotherapy department did little to help apart from their initial assessment. After returning home he fell again twice and then was admitted once again to Torbay Hospital. Realising that Gerald had little hope of recovering his balance or being able to walk again he was placed in Woodrow Retirement home where he is now being cared for with great kindness 24 hours a day and I am grateful to Social Services for their help in this ideal placement.

Chapter 3

Care Villages

Care Villages are now being provided in many parts of the country and I do recommend inspection visits to as many as possible as they usually have their own particular specialities and should provide facilities for both carer and cared-for. I have visited several Care Villages, particularly along the south coast. The first phases of St. George's Park at Ditchling, Sussex are virtually complete. The Sunrise Senior Living Developments in Eastbourne, Southampton and Dorset are opening their doors and Audley are already welcoming their first guests at the Mote House near Maidstone. These developments cater for dementia patients in specialist accommodation and also offer flats of various sizes for retirement living. They all offer transport to the local towns as well as providing shops and restaurants on site and provide Home Care. However I was disappointed that St. George's Park did not offer Day Care activity in the village nursing home.

I particularly liked the security of the 'package of care' that Richmond Care Villages offer their residents

– particularly the 2am 'tiptoe in' visit to ensure that everyone is safely tucked-up in bed – very reassuring!

Care Villages are rapidly spreading throughout England and offer a much higher standard of care than the past run of the mill 'being put in a home' atmosphere where the odour of boiled cabbage and urine soaked carpets leave a lasting memory of your visit.

The cost of social care for the growing population of elderly and mentally ill is a major problem, purely because there is no money in the national budget to care for them!

Over many years different Governments have radically changed their attitudes to caring. Gone are the Victorian institutions to be replaced by 'Care in the Community.' Neither system, in my opinion, is the kindest or the best for the patients or their families. Units built solely and specifically as E.M. I. Units can never improve the quality of life for the patients. Imagine if you will a 80 year old woman in the early to mid stages of Dementia who has no other way of spending her days except seated in a crowded room surrounded by others who are likely to be in their later stages of the illness, moaning and shouting. The television is switched on and the sound is either off or on full blast. The smell of the urine soaked carpet pervades the room and the windows are usually tight shut. Although there is a garden no one goes out into it, except on the day of the annual fund raising garden party when it usually rains!

Homes are short staffed. The Fillipino carers work hard, although they struggle to understand the residents, and the residents give up trying to understand the carers.

As the patients have difficulty eating the food is cheap, overcooked and often tastes of freezer-burn.

Imagine that same woman in the comfort of her own room with her own furniture and television, able to walk out and sit in the garden, visited by a chiropodist, occupational therapist, physiotherapist and a hairdresser. The carers are English and are qualified; they consult her on her likes and dislikes and she is served afternoon tea with homemade cakes and is able to choose from a varied supper menu. Is this too much to ask? Is it too much to ask that patients can have privacy and dignity and be served with a choice of food?

The choice of moving into a Nursing Home, a Retirement Home, or a Care Village will depend on your state of health, and whether you prefer independence; or whether your need for care is such that it dictates dependence on nursing care.

A check list of facilities and services when taking a look at Care Villages:
1. Are you able to sell your present home and buy a property in the care village?

You need to take into account future maintenance fees which may increase annually, Stamp Duty, costs of removal, Solicitors and Estate Agents fees, and HIP. (Home Information Pack) If your present home takes a long time to sell you may be faced with negotiating a 'bridging loan' or reducing your 'asking price'. Some homes encourage you to rent your chosen property for two years in order to give you time to sell your own home.

2. Does the home provide Day Care on site?

If there is no Day Care you may both end up incarcerated in a small apartment 24 hours a day. Day Care facilities, either on site or in a near-by town are essential

3. Is the living accommodation spacious enough to accommodate your own favourite pieces of furniture and kitchen equipment?

You need to be happy in your surroundings.

4. Will you be within reasonable driving distance of friends and family?

It's a mistake to lose touch.

5. Will my pets be allowed?
If not you'll miss them terribly.

6. Will the management of your new home assist with your removals?

With the present economic situation many retirement villages now offer this facility.

7. Does the management offer transport facilities into near-by towns for Medical and Dental appointments, shopping, concerts etc. and is there a hairdresser, restaurant and shop on site?

This is essential if you don't have your own car.

Chapter 4

Continuing Care...
From Cradle to Grave?

When the NHS was introduced that is what we were promised – Care from Cradle to Grave. There was no warning that care depended on means testing for the elderly and handicapped. Although treatment, prescriptions for pensioners, medication and medical and surgical procedures are available free of charge on the NHS, nowadays no one is entitled to funding for home care, residential and nursing home care unless their savings and income are below £23,250 per year or their medical condition is so serious that nursing care is essential throughout the day or night.

Long term funding for Continuing Care can be provided by the NHS, or by Social Services as 'Social Care,' provided that the patient's savings and income are below the 'means test' level set by the Government, and they are based on a sliding scale.

'**Social Care**' usually includes washing, bathing, dressing, toileting and personal care as well as feeding, shopping, cleaning and the administration of medication; which can be provided at home or in a residential or nursing home.

'**Nursing Care**' does not depend on a patient's savings and income but on the mental and physical condition of the patient's health.

The patient's state of health is judged by eleven Decision Support Tools known as Domains and each domain is sub divided into statements of need i.e. No needs, Low, Moderate, High, Severe or Priority levels of need, depending on the domain.

The domains are classified as :

Behaviour;   Cognitive Impairment, Psychological & Emotional, Communication, Mobility, Nutrition, Continence, Skin and Tissue Viability, Breathing, Drug Therapy and Medication, and Altered States of Consciousness.

These Decision Support Tools and Needs Assessment will be explained in detail as an appendix at the end of the book and it is vitally important to understand them and use them.

If you decide to apply to the Primary Care Trust (PCT) for Continuing Care Funding the patient will need to be assessed on his or her needs. The assessment will be carried out by a member of staff of the Primary Care Trust, usually a Community Psychiatric Nurse (CPN) who will make a recommendation to a Panel that will consider the application.

Following Gerald's diagnosis his condition deteriorated and I was lucky to be given plenty of advice from Torbay Social Services. After a further two years I was advised to apply for Funding for Continuing Care. I was told that the procedure was likely to drag on for as long as four years or more before I would be successful and that the sooner I started the better. How right they were! We are now approaching crisis point with Gerald's condition, the country is also in an economic crisis and the Government is reluctant to provide financial assistance for the elderly, sick and disabled.

Although I made two applications to the PCT, on each occasion I was never shown a copy of the criteria so it was impossible for me to know what the Trust's criteria actually was.

On the first occasion the application was submitted by the Community Psychiatric Nurse (CPN) and I had very little input. Eventually I was sent a copy which enabled me to tailor the application to meet their requirements and I was also fortunate to be offered help by Mike Pearce, an adviser from the Alzheimer's Society, whose advice was invaluable. After some months the PCT offered me the opportunity to appeal to an 'Independent Panel' set up by the PCT and Mike assisted me with my written presentation.

My daughter accompanied me to the hearing giving me moral support and verifying my evidence, we had a full and fair hearing despite the fact that some members had past links with the PCT. I also gained the impression that the appeal panel members had already been told by the PCT that even if they did agree to my application there was no money in their budget to fund it. This opinion was confirmed when at a later date I enquired when I would be informed of the panel's decision. I was told that it would take some time as the panel was arranging a meeting with the PCT to discuss the case! (Rather like a judge discussing the case with the prosecution before announcing his verdict.)

Some weeks later I received the decision *"We recognise that Mr. Hill has needs over a number of care domains but they are not of such complexity for the panel to recommend Continuing Health Care."*

Once again I was asked if I disagreed with the decision and wished to take the matter further. Of course I did!

Luckily, about this time, I came across an advertisement, in a weekend newspaper, from an organisation called Cheselden Continuing Care . *'If you are paying for Continuing Care you may qualify for NHS funding.'* I didn't waste time - I send them full details of the situation. After some further correspondence they agreed to represent us and I signed an agreement on a 'no win no fee' basis – in other words - when we won the case I would keep 70% of the reimbursement and send Cheselden 30%.

At the end of November 2008 I drove to Exeter to present my case to the South West Regional Health Authority. Colin Ball, from Cheselden Continuing Care, also drove down from Wilmslow to provide moral support and act as an observer. We had a fair hearing from a panel who were truly independent. I was told that we would hear the result in 5 weeks time. What sort of a Christmas Present would that prove to be?

Christmas passed and so did New Year. In mid January I telephoned the South West Regional Health Authority to ask when I could expect to receive the result. "Before the end of the month." was the reply. As I sit here composing my first draft it is now February – and still nothing. Once again I telephoned, and this time I was told that I would receive the result "within two weeks," which takes us to the third week in February which will be three months after the appeal to the SW Strategic Health Authority (SW SHA).

Again at the end of February I wrote to the SW SHA and informed them that unless they sent me the panel's decision within seven working days I would register a formal complaint against them. They replied immediately that they would meet my 'timetable.'

Today is the 3rd. of March, the sixth working day, and I spoke to the SW SHA who assured me that the reply was 'going through the system!' The department seemed surprised that we had now reached the sixth working day, but promised that once the letter was signed by the Chief Executive it would be posted and e-mailed to me. He also assured me that such delays were normal!

Next day I posted my formal letter of complaint. On 11th of March I received a long letter from the Chairman of the South West Regional Health Authority informing me (in Civil Service jargon) that we had been granted funding for Continuing Care. In simple terms I had won!

Chapter 5

Financial Matters

Should my appeal have failed Cheselden had already examined all the accounts and receipts   sent to me from Torbay Council in order to prepare a claim against them on my behalf.

Means Testing. Social Care has to be paid for unless capital and income are below the 'means test' level and this applies no matter whether the patient is cared for in his own home or in a residential or nursing home.

A complex assessment of capital, income and expenditure has to be worked out. For example, how much do you as a carer or spouse need to budget for Council Tax, mortgage, rent and maintenance costs on your property, water rates, gas and electricity, transport, clothing, insurance and food for all the family and pets. How much does it cost to run the car or take a holiday ?

Thousands of elderly people are being forced to sell their homes in order to pay care home fees and many councils fail to observe the guidelines that state that pensioners can retain their family home if another elderly relative is living there. As a result many people are not informed of their rights and entitlements.

The law states that if an elderly person holds more than £23,250 in capital they are expected to pay the full cost of care. This includes the value of any property as well as savings and investments, but in certain circumstances, where a patient is going into a care home who has a spouse, a relative aged over 60 years old, or younger than 16, or a relative on incapacity benefit living with them their property is automatically exempted from the means test.

There are other ways to protect a person's capital, such as placing assets in trusts for relatives, but this needs to be arranged at an early stage, well before the need for care arises in order to avoid being accused of 'deliberate deprivation.' If the local authority believes that assets have been given away, specifically to avoid paying care costs they have the legal right to challenge these disposals and to grab these funds.

Age Concern has already warned that "where a disposal of assets is treated as deliberate deprivation, the local authority will include 'notional capital' to the value of those assets in its assessment of your means."

Those wishing to protect their assets should consider splitting joint accounts. By doing this only the savings of the patient who is entering the care home would be eroded and the council would help with fees once those assets fall below £23,250.

Certain investments are also excluded from the local authority's means test. This includes investment bonds which contain an element of life assurance.

It is important that investors have a genuine financial reason for taking out such a bond, otherwise a sudden switch from Isas into investment bonds could also be counted as deliberate deprivation.

It is therefore essential that anyone who is applying for funding for continuing care should always seek specialist financial advice at the earliest possible moment.

The Finance and Benefits team (FAB) of your local council – if they play fair – should give you honest advice, but you also need to get advice from a reputable financial adviser as you will need to take into account Inheritance Tax planning and Capital Gains Tax issues and at the same time safeguard your own income

The Health Service Ombudsman

If you have been unreasonably refused an Independent Review, or if you are not satisfied with the outcome of an Independent Review you can take your case to the Health Service Ombudsman and you should do this within one year from the date you became aware of the issue.

However if you have commenced legal action or intend to sue, the Ombudsman will not investigate your complaint.

Contact www.ombudsman.org.uk
Telephone: 0845 015 4033

Chapter 6

Coping with Crises

Patients with dementia often exhibit different and changeable behaviour, no two are alike. As time passes it becomes almost impossible to cope with the change that is taking place. Gerald had always been calm and had a pleasant nature. Usually he was an extraordinarily patient man but within months everything had changed. The man I married was no longer there, instead he had turned into someone else, someone who handed you a saucer when you asked him for his cup, someone who put his shoes on the wrong feet and walked out of the front door when he needed to go to the toilet. He would walk into other people's flats, put his clothes on over his pyjamas and sometimes try to put on my clothes instead of his own. To begin with I would say "Don't be silly. Think what you are doing."

I tried to bring him to his senses, I shouted, became impatient and angry at such stupidity. It was a particularly bad time for both of us. I was advised to walk away into another room when he became aggressive; but you can't do that when you are driving the car and he continually fiddles with the controls, or when he throws his food onto the floor and the gravy congeals on the carpet and he blames you for causing the mess.

The most distressing problem is incontinence, especially when someone is doubly incontinent. Washing clothes, carpets, upholstery and beds, bathing and showering can be exhausting and embarrassing both for the sufferer and the carer. One evening it took me five hours to clean up the flat after a particularly horrifying occasion when he walked around naked, emptying his bowels as he shuffled through the lounge.

The most important action you can take is to contact the Continence Service, through your GP. The patient has to be assessed and the service will normally provide Continence Pads. You will need to discuss the size of the pads – the smaller pads are for urinary incontinence, but an adult who is doubly incontinent will require a much larger size. Don't accept the first type that is sent to you if it is not suitable, you can always change the type of pad. If the person gets upset at the thought of wearing a pad you may wish to consider using the Home Care service to come in and help. You and your GP will also need to consider whether a change of medication or diet has caused the problem. In our case the consultant described the problem as 'cognitive.'

You may also find that the quiet, gentle person who you fell in love with becomes verbally and physically aggressive, they may take to alcohol, become unable to hold a conversation, unable to find their way in the house, unable to dress themselves and become totally confused.

You will not be alone! You will discover that in your town the Mental Health Team hold regular meetings for carers to discuss their problems and get advice on how to cope. If you register as a Carer and take part in all the ongoing activities of the group you will benefit enormously from their help and support.

However if you, like me, want to get away and have some relief from the pressures of coping then do as I do and take the dog for a walk!

Living with Alzheimers means continual problem solving, as soon as one problem is solved another one arises.

As the years passed his condition deteriorated. He lost all short term memory, became almost totally blind, refused to eat – except for chocolate and cake – and became an alcoholic which aggravated his confusion and his incontinence. He no longer has spells of clarity. He has unexpected spells of breathlessness, hyperventilation and chest pains and a racing pulse. The first few times I called the ambulance and he was admitted to hospital. Now these incidents happen so often that I wait for them to pass - usually about an hour - as going into hospital causes him distress and after all it is better than catching MRSA! He can barely shuffle and has frequent falls, resulting in cuts and bruises. He also has cellulitis and swollen legs and ankles.

As his condition worsened I became more and more distraught and began using swear words that I did not even know that I knew! Social Services recommended that I should attend a course of Counselling sessions, but that didn't help at all. Being so short of time to myself I preferred to take my dog a walk on the beach rather than spend several hours a week discussing my relationship with my husband. The Counsellor also suggested that if I wanted more time to myself I should give up playing bowls – that suggestion annoyed me as I really did enjoy a game of bowls! After crashing my car and near to losing my self-control my G.P. sympathetically prescribed a non-addictive anti-depressant called Citalopram. Then things really looked up. I stopped swearing and began to smile and my sense of humour returned. Gerald went into care and I took several short holidays. I was relieved to discover that I enjoyed my own company and was not at all fazed at being an independent traveller.

I solved the alcohol problem by diluting the wine and spirits half and half which he does not notice as he had lost his taste. Luckily he still enjoys soup and I make plenty of that.

He spent two days a week with his host carer and two days a week at day-care which meant that I had time to myself out in the fresh air playing bowls.

Some months ago another new problem began, his nose began to run continuously. He could not tell that it was happening and it was worse at the start of every meal when it streamed down the front of his clothes. Then he begins to sneeze so violently that it made his nose bleed. I had to make him lie down on the sofa and pack his nostrils with cotton wool, but then he sneezed again and blew out the cotton wool. Another major cleaning job!

I have now discovered a decorative chain from 'Scotts of Stowe' that will go around his neck and has two clasps that clip on to a serviette that lies across his chest. So much nicer than a plastic bib or apron!

Last winter proved difficult for Gerald as he feels the cold very badly. The winter fuel payment did little to meet the high electricity costs and he put on extra layers of clothes. He constantly fiddles with the thermostat which is always on maximum and when I left him to go shopping he went around the flat turning switches on and off and trying to put in extra plugs. The result? I found him in the dark, having 'blown' the trip switch! He constantly switches on all the lights – I have had 'timer' switches fitted on many lights and taped over other switches, especially in the kitchen. When we are in the car he fiddles with all the buttons and switches, then I have to stop the car and threaten to take him back home.

He seems to have taken an active dislike to soap and water and taking a bath. He is supposed to be bathed at day-care, but recently he has refused to co-operate. Until then he always co-operated with male carers, especially if they wore uniform, but now when I call in a male carer to bathe him at home he swears and struggles to get out of the bath.

There may be many occasions when you and the patient have disagreements. I found that aggression for both of us usually happened when dressing, undressing and bathing. When my G.P. prescribed anti-depressants for me the result was very effective – I became pleasant and reasonable, working out how to avoid difficulties and as a result Gerald also became much more amenable – he still dislikes soap and water but I learned to humour him and generally succeeded in my efforts.

Chapter 7

Benefits and Power of Attorney

Power of Attorney

The time will eventually come for everyone when they can no longer manage their own affairs, maybe through blindness, dementia or other illness and it is a good idea to address this problem well before it is really necessary. In our case we arranged an appointment with our solicitor and made the necessary arrangements. Gradually as his illness progressed I took over Gerald's financial affairs, signing cheques and using Microsoft Money to record his accounts on the computer. I found it useful to keep several copies of the Enduring Power of Attorney to send to the bank and other organisations in order to prove that I was legally acting on his behalf. This worked well. Recently I applied to register my Enduring Power of Attorney with the **'Public Guardian'** as Gerald's mental state had deteriorated so badly that he failed to understand what was happening.

I found the Office of the Public Guardian very helpful. Their web site is www.publicguardian.gov.uk and their phone number is **0845 330 2900**

It is always a good idea to keep other members of the family in touch with the situation and I also keep a record of all transactions on the computer, then if questions should be asked, I can print off information. From time to time I am asked questions by the local authority about our capital and income and it is always wise to be completely open and helpful when discussing such matters with those who have the authority to ask.

Attendance Allowance

Attendance Allowance is a tax free benefit for people aged 65 or over who have an illness or disability and need help with personal care. It is not normally affected by savings or any other income. There are two rates, the lower rate for those who needs care during the day and the higher rate for those who need care during the day and night. I have had no difficulty in obtaining Attendance Allowance at the higher rate for my husband. The amount is paid monthly and although it will not in any way meet the full cost of paying for all your needs it does at least help in a small way.

Carer's Allowance

If you are claiming Attendance Allowance and there is someone looking after you for 35 hours or more a week they may be able to get Carer's Allowance. However if that person is already receiving a pension or other state benefit they will not be able to claim Carer's Allowance as they may lose their right to receive their existing benefit. It seems hard that a pensioner cannot claim Carer's Allowance!

For further information on Attendance Allowance and Carer's Allowance contact Social Services or the Department of Work and Pensions on 01253 856123 – but please bear in mind that though this information is correct at the time of writing, the Government is continually reviewing its policies about care of the elderly and the regulations can, and probably will, change.

Council Tax benefits

Sufferers from Dementia can apply for a **Status Discount for the Severely Mentally Impaired**. Amongst the conditions that have to be met are that the sufferer is entitled to Attendance Allowance. If you satisfy the conditions you will receive a discount on your Council Tax.

Registered blind?

You may also be eligible for a discount if you set aside a room in your home for your Merlin Reader, Talking Book CD player, or your computer which is equipped with Zoom Text, in fact any gadget or machine that helps you to read or write – especially machines that read text.

Lifeline Alarm System

Your local council may provide a Lifeline Alarm System which gives carers peace of mind if they have to leave home for a short while to go shopping. The alarm provides a voice link between your home and the Council's alarm centre 24 hours a day, every day of the year, and works even in another room, bedroom, bathroom or toilet.

The alarm works through your telephone system when you press a pendant that you can wear either around your wrist, like a watch, or around your neck. This sends a signal down the telephone line to the alarm centre and will automatically tell the staff who the call is from. You can then tell the operator about the problem. If however you do not speak the operator will then treat the call as urgent and contact the emergency services.

Lifeline can also be used to answer the phone without getting up from your chair to use the hand set. For more information contact your local authority Social Services department.

If you are partially sighted **Doro Mobile Phones** are now producing an 'easy to use' mobile phone suitable for elderly people who have poor sight. Their phone number is **08450111160** and they can also be contacted by e-mail on: www.easytousemobiles.com or by Google on Doro mobile phones.

Another useful aid is a P**ressure pad** placed on a chair beneath the sufferer which emits a loud 'bleep' to alert the carer if a patient who is likely to fall tries to get out of their chair.

Most Social Service Departments will loan equipment such as pressure pads, Zimmer Frames, Three Wheel Walkers and raised Toilet Seats with arms and it is worthwhile discussing your needs with Social Services.

Chapter 8

Carers and Caring

If you wish to care for your relative or a patient at home you will need help. In the later stages of the illness you will certainly be unable to manage on your own. It will be a demanding full time job and you will need time off to go shopping, have some social life and take an occasional break. Who will be ready to step in if you are taken ill or need a holiday? The costs of Home Care are high £14 to £18 per hour depending which part of the country you live in and it can easily exceed the costs of a nursing home. Those of us who saved and paid into occupational pensions now find that we just cannot afford to pay for care in our old age and the State cannot afford to do so either. Unless we pay very much more into our private pensions and unless the state introduces new schemes to care for the elderly and disabled the future becomes increasingly bleak year by year.

During the three years that I have felt it necessary to employ Home Care I have increased the number of days and hours for Gerald's sake and also for my sake. At the beginning his Key Worker contacted **Age Concern** to see if they could arrange to set up one day a week for him in their **Host Carer scheme**. Host Carers welcome elderly, and disabled people into their homes for one or two days a week. They try to arrange for a group of like-minded people to get together each day. In Gerald's case, his Host Carer has several ex-servicemen, who have much to reminisce about. If the weather is nice they go out for coffee or visit a garden-centre. As time passed his condition got worse and it was suggested that he should spend two days a week with Eleanor his Host Carer. He was always very happy to see her when she came for him in her own car. Eleanor had the warmth and love that is typical of an Irish woman and is so appreciated by people who are disabled.

Within weeks he became unable to get in and out of the bath so Claire, his Key Worker, arranged for him to be collected twice a week to go to Day Care at Eclipse Lodge, a residential home for patients with dementia who also cater for Day Care patients. I found it a useful arrangement as he was bathed and his legs, that were affected by cellulitis, were also treated. The home offered a regular programme of activities that included quizzes, reminiscence groups, music and singing and the staff were loving and sympathetic. Sometimes if I needed to take a break Gerald would stay either at Eclipse Lodge or with Eleanor and he seemed happy to stay at either home. I really believe that we were lucky to find these two solutions.

When Gerald became doubly incontinent he seemed embarrassed that I should change his soiled pads and deal with his personal hygiene so after continual bouts of aggression in the evening it was decided that an organisation called Homecare 2000 should be asked to send in male carers to get him ready for bed. This works well and we are both able to go to bed in a calm atmosphere. He is washed and has his teeth cleaned as well as Listerine mouth wash which is essential as he has lost many teeth and the roots, which are still in place, would become infected if it were not for the mouthwash. He is not fit enough to undergo surgery to remove the roots with a general anaesthetic. The reason for losing his teeth is that he has difficulty with swallowing and chewed up his tablets which caused his teeth to rot.

Gerald is doubly incontinent and frequently opens his bowels wherever he is. We do have a continence clinic in Newton Abbot who supply continence pads, but I have a problem getting them to understand the type and size of pads that are needed. Although I have asked for this situation to be monitored the District Nurses who run the service are so short of staff that no one ever visits to assess whether the service that they provide is effective and necessary. So far it has taken nearly three years to get suitable equipment although I am told that there is even better equipment available.

Chapter 9

Success!

The decision I had waited for so long was dated December 2008 and told me that the panel had unanimously agreed that Gerald was eligible for Continuing Care funding!

I then wrote to the Chief Executive of the SW SHA to formally complain about the length of time it had taken to send me the decision. In his reply the Chief Executive described the delay as 'unreasonable' and assured me that he would set up an inquiry and let me know the outcome before the end of the month.

As far as I was concerned the reasons for the panel's decision were clearly understandable. The panel members accepted the primary health care arguments and also considered whether the Grogan Judgement applied in this case. The panel unanimously concluded that my husband did meet the criteria for NHS Funded Continuing Care and also recommended that Torbay Care Trust should carry out a fresh joint care needs assessment, given the evidence of his changing needs and condition.

My own advice which may be useful to all those who are battling for Funding for NHS Continuing Care is as follows:

Be calm and completely determined to win.

Do not be put off. (Several staff from Torbay Trust visited me and did their best to persuade me to give up the fight).

Study previous judgements such as Coughlin, Grogan and previous Ombudsman cases.

Study newspaper reports.

Keep detailed records of conversations and letters and build up a file

Keep notes of all medications.

Ask for copies of admission reports, ward reports and hospital notes and record the names of all NHS staff who visit you.

Remember to record the dates and the name of the ward, also the name of the medical staff.

Keep daily notes of all incidents and the health of the patient.

Write up your notes legibly at the end of the day.

Do not be afraid to make use of the local and national press..

Legal Advice.

There are many solicitors who would be happy to advise you and represent you at a hearing of the Primary Care Trust, or the Strategic Health Authority, but solicitor's fees are expensive and the case can drag on for several years. I was lucky to find Cheselden Continuing Care and I signed an agreement to pay them 30% of any money I received in compensation. In effect it was a 'no win-no fee' agreement. Having read the papers that I sent them they told me that I had a good case and that they would represent me. Although I actually presented the case to the panel the Cheselden advice was invaluable.

Equally invaluable was the advice I received from Mike Pearce from the Alzheimers Society. With his great experience he knew exactly how the papers should be written. Without Mike's advice I would never have had the confidence and knowledge to argue so forcibly with the Primary Care Trust or the Strategic Health Authority. I wrote, amended and revised my case for presentation many times e-mailing it to Mike, often receiving the corrections back the same day. From start to finish the whole procedure took three years; many others took far longer. Many solicitors do not have the experience to handle these sort of cases, nor have they studied the appeals procedure or judgements in the High Court so it is important to search for an experienced legal adviser before committing yourself to great expense.

Chapter 10

Falls and other crises

'It's an ill wind…'

Following the arrival of the good news, two months later at the end of April 2009 Gerald tried to get up from his chair, lost his balance and fell awkwardly. He was obviously in great pain and I phoned for the ambulance who took him to the hospital where they told me that he had broken his hip. He had a total hip replacement and after five days was transferred to a convalescent unit at Paignton Hospital. The surgery was totally successful, but despite my efforts to encourage the Physiotherapy Department to treat him with post operative exercises and help him to use his walking frame Gerald became weaker, lost his balance several times and also lost confidence in his ability to ever walk again. He was eventually discharged from hospital and sent home. Next morning he refused to get out of bed or try to walk to the toilet so the ambulance returned and took him back to hospital.

Later that day he came home once again. I settled him in his arm chair and he asked for some supper. As I left the room to go to the kitchen I heard him shout – I turned back and found him on the floor, bleeding from his head. He had left his chair and fallen and hit his forehead on the fireplace!

Eventually after further assessment in hospital it was decided that as he was so frail and unable to stand or walk he should be should go into a nursing home. Claire Rowland, his key worker, arranged for him to go to a retirement home close to where we live. I took the family to have a look at it and we were all delighted with the facilities. It had everything that Gerald needed, including kind-hearted, thoughtful staff and very good food – a place where the individual patient was catered for and came first.

The patients were elderly, some had early dementia but most enjoyed conversation, good food and had a good quality of life. Daily life was quiet and peaceful and we all hoped that from now on his problems were temporarily at an end.

APPENDIX 1

Continuing Care

APPEAL

1. *Document Purpose*

The purpose of this document is to clearly show that both the physical and mental health of Mr. Gerald Hill has deteriorated so as to justify the granting of continuous care funding for his care at his home address.

This document is submitted by Mrs. Jane Hill on behalf of Gerald Hill for the purpose of the review to be undertaken by Torbay PCT, or S.W. Strategic Health Authority, and should be read in conjunction with PCT assessments, hospital and GP records to show his current condition.

2. *Brief History*

Gerald Hill is 88 years of age, born on 6/1/1921 in Nantwich, Cheshire. He retired from his practice as a solicitor due to ill health in 1988 . In World War 2 he served in the RNVR on Russian Convoys and on D Day he captained a Tank Landing Craft in the spear head of the landings. In 1945 he served in operations in Java and other sectors in the Far East.

At the onset of his present illness in 2000 we sold our house in Cheshire and moved to our current address, as Gerald had by then become unable to cope with the property.

His present condition is briefly summarised as:

Communication – Unable to converse for more than a very short period of time on any subject or to describe his discomfort.

Cognitive impairment – Unable to make decisions. Disorientated, confused. Almost completely blind. Marked short term memory impairment (limited to seconds) Unable to assess risks. Gets lost.

M*obility* –Before his accident he could only shuffle a short distance and had daily falls resulting in bruising and bleeding. Following a fall at the end of October he could only stumble in a disorientated manner. However **since he broke his hip in April he is unable to walk without a walking frame and the assistance of at least one member of staff.**

Doubly incontinent – Continual and complete loss of bodily control

Skin Care – Skin described as 'paper thin,' resulting in Cellulitis. Legs and ankles are very swollen.

Nutrition – Dysphagia..Has difficulty in eating and often refuses to eat. Reliant on 'Ensure.' Severe and continuing weight loss

Behaviour – At home he had challenging and unpredictable aggression, lashing out and hitting his wife over the head and face, swearing loudly and banging the furniture.

Breathing At home - shortness of breath. Hyperventilation and panting resulting in racing pulse rate. Frequent chest pains and tachycardia. Shortness of breath. Since he has been at Woodrow Retirement Home this problem has lessened.

Emotional and Psychological – Unable to engage in a care plan or daily activities. Appears distressed and confused. Loses his way in the flat. Behaves like a 2 year old child. Appears seriously depressed.

Medical History

1970 *Aged 49* – Heart Attack. Treated at Mid Cheshire Hospital, Crewe.

1980 *Aged 59* – TIA. Treated at Manchester PPH (Dr Lascelles)

1998 *Aged 77* – Hypertension. Duodenal Ulcer, Oesophagitis. TIAs.

2001 Aged 80 - Macular Degeneration, Amaurosis Fugax, Glaucoma, , Diaphragmatic Hernia, Treated at Mid Cheshire Hospital, Crewe. (Dr. Neugebaur)

2002 *Aged 81* – Polymyalgia Rheumatica, Mid Cheshire Hospital, Crewe. (Dr Mackay)

2003 Aged 82 –Registered blind. Adnocarcinoma of Prostate – TURP, Mount Stewart Hospital, 2 weeks, (Mr. Seamus Mcdermott)

2004 *Aged 83* – Diagnosed Alzheimers disease, Chadwell Centre, Dr.Somerfield.

2005 *Aged 85* - Impaired kidney function, Shortage of breath, Low Blood Pressure, Tachycardia, Chest pains. Admitted to Torbay Hospital, 2 weeks. (Dr Uridge)

2007 *Aged 86* – Cellulitis, Urinary Tract Infection, Toxic confusion.

Admitted to Torbay Hospital, (Simpson Ward) 1 week. Dr. Sinclair, Mr. S.A.Cope.

Dysphagia, Doubly incontinent, Aggressive, Total Loss of bodily control.

Decision Support Tool details

BEHAVIOUR
Severe
Challenging behaviour of severity and frequency that presents an immediate and serious risk to self or others. The risks are so serious that any response could well be outside the range of planned intervention. As his carer I am constantly at risk

At home Gerald frequently lost his temper and became violent and aggressive whenever he was asked to do something (eat food, co-operate with his dressing etc). His aggression was unpredictable, noisy and violent, shouting and swearing and happened most days. Our daily rows were frightening and I had to physically restrain him by pushing him down on to a chair. He was particularly aggressive whenever I tried to carry out personal hygiene and change his pads. When I put on his clean pad he threw his soiled pad directly at my face and swore and hit me across the head. As he would not wash or use soap I had difficulty in keeping him clean, so he was bathed twice a week at Eclipse Lodge.. He also suffered from depression and during the day sits for long periods in brooding silence or sighing. If people ask him how he is he usually shouts at them, telling them that he cannot see. (See notes made by William Tabron CPN referring to his aggression in December 2006)

Since **June 2008** I arranged for a carer to come in the evening to help Gerald get ready for bed, undressing him, changing his pad and putting on his pyjamas. For a few days all went well and there were no evening rows. However he then countered this plan by waiting for the carer to depart, then when I was busy elsewhere he would shuffle into the bedroom, strip off his pyjamas and continence pad, leaving them on the floor, and stumble around naked. Then I had to go through the whole procedure of putting on a clean pad and his pyjamas, and the aggression and the noise was worse than ever. The number of times when he tried to undress himself is now increasing.

December 2008 Gerald is now refusing to be bathed at Eclipse Lodge and I have to ask the carers who come in during the evening if they will bath him. This causes noisy rows and much swearing "I'm not getting in the bloody bath!"

He has now become alcohol dependent and tries to get into the kitchen and mix drinks at all times of the day. He is unable to identify the bottles and pours anything he can find into his glass.

Recently one afternoon I went out to the local shops. When I returned several parts of the flat were in darkness. Gerald had tried to turn on the radiator, then tried to plug in several wall lights and eventually had 'blown' the trip switch. Even when I take him out in the car he continually presses the switches and dials on the dashboard. He is a constant liability and it is risky to leave him alone. Although he can hardly walk he does manage to shuffle out of the flat and gets lost and often wanders into another person's flat and falls down.

His Behaviour can only be classed as Severe (rather than Moderate)

COGNITION
Severe
Severe cognitive impairment which is likely to include marked short term and long term memory issues and disorientation in time and place. The individual is unable to assess basic risks and is dependent on others to protect them from harm. Severely disorientated.

Gerald is now very disorientated, and this condition is aggravated by macular degeneration. He is unaware of his bodily functions and regularly evacuates his bowels wherever he is. Whilst at his Host Carer's home he did this and she had to throw all his clothes away as they were too badly soiled to wash. He is completely unaware of his incontinence, and often walks through his excreta and treads it throughout the flat, or tries to go to bed in soiled pyjamas.

There is a severe risk of recurring infection due to faeces coating his legs and coming in contact with the badly damaged skin on his legs. (He has already spent a week in hospital with cellulitis and toxic confusion as a result of the skin on his legs breaking down).

I do need however to address this problem under the heading of Continence –

He does not know where he is outside his home, he cannot identify every day items in the house e.g. differentiate between a cup and a saucer, he is unable to operate a switch, although he constantly tries to do so and puts himself at risk. Plugs and switches have to be taped up as a protection and some essential switches have now been fitted with timers. He needs to be constantly supervised as he is a danger to himself.

In addition he cannot make decisions. He does not know the day of the week, or the time of day, he does not know whether he has had a meal, he is completely unable to take part in a conversation, his memory loss is severe as he immediately forgets every word that is said to him within seconds. He cannot read, he is unable to understand RNIB Talking Books.

He is seriously disorientated and several times has wandered off into other people's flats and has to be brought home. He is very confused and since his operation in April 2009 he has lost the use of his legs. It should be recognised that a male carer is present for half an hour in the evening whilst I am with Gerald for the remaining twenty three and a half hours. He now appears to have forgotten how to open a door by turning the door handle, so he and rattles and bangs doors – especially the lavatory door- which aggravates his incontinence problems and his anger. Unfortunately the front door is easily opened as a fire exit.

His condition should be classified as Severe (rather than High)

PSYCHOLOGICAL & EMOTIONAL NEEDS
High

Requires prompts to engage in care plan and demonstrates difficulty in engaging in care plan and or daily activities. Anxiety symptoms that impact on an individual's health or well being. Withdraws from attempts to engage them in support/care planning.

Due to his various illnesses, dementia and blindness, Gerald has difficulty in engaging in most activities.

He has periods of depression, appears distressed and lost, continually moans and sighs and grimaces, pulling faces as if in pain.. At home he was alcohol dependent but now, as he is unable to walk, the staff control his alcohol intake.

He has been diagnosed as having Toxic Confusion as a result of Cellulitis.

He requires assistance throughout the day

He has unpredictable mood changes which are marked by aggression and violence in the presence of his carer (myself) but can quickly change in the presence of visitors or his male nurse. However he is regularly uncooperative (due to inability to remember what they have told him) He is very confused and cannot understand what I tell him.

The panel classified this as High

MOBILITY

High

High risk of falls.

Prior to April 2009 Gerald was unsteady, lost his balance and frequently fell. He fells down several times a week and I am not able to help him get up. His face is often bruised and bleeding and he has to crawl to a chair or his bed and with my help get to his feet. Gerald will never leave his chair unless urged or prompted – even for a meal and he prefers to sleep all day in one position. In the apartment he stumbles and outside he has to use a wheelchair if we have to walk any distance. Oedema. His legs and ankles are very swollen and he needs extra large footwear.

At the October panel my husband's mobility was classified as Moderate. This is inaccurate as there is ample evidence to show that he is at high risk of falls. **However the recent July panel did classify it as High.**

The Assessment Tool for Patients at Risk of Falling used on 27/02/05 in Torbay Hospital Emergency Room *classified him as 13/15, i.e. at <u>Very High Risk</u>. Again on 22/2/07, the* Patient Risk Assessment Tool Review Record, *states '<u>High falls risk, confused</u>'.* Following a fall in October his mobility has further deteriorated. He is in pain and until April was only able to stumble from chair to chair. Since April, when he fell and broke his hip, he has been totally immobile without assistance and his walking frame. He has been classified as being at very high risk of falls. <u>On 13th August the Head of Physiotherapy visited me to tell me that that despite all the efforts of the physiotherapy team there was no hope of Gerald ever being able to walk again. His brain had now lost control of his legs.</u>

<u>Therefore Mr Hill's mobility needs should be classified as High</u>.

NUTRITION

High

Dysphagia. Unintended significant weight loss. Nutritional status "at risk."

Gerald suffers from Dysphagia. A spoonful of soup takes five minutes to swallow – even a spoonful of thin soup has to be chewed for 5 minutes before he is able to swallow. Every mouthful of food has to be chewed continuously before he can manage to swallow it and the food goes cold

He regularly refuses to use a knife, spoon or fork

Mealtimes occupy most of the day

Most meals are replaced by 'Ensure' (prescribed by the GP) I do not recall the GP telling me not to worry! In fact at a Review meeting with Dr David Somerfield, Consultant, on 18th. January 2009 Dr Somerfield noticed that Gerald was very weak and needed more calories in his diet. I explained that Gerald eats very little and Dr Somerfield recommended dietary supplements and that he should be weighed weekly. His weight loss is significant and very noticeable and he is losing weight rapidly. Most days he refuses to eat, even if he is assisted

He picks up his food in his fingers and drops it on the carpet for the dog

When faced with food his nose runs and he starts to sneeze violently. This causes his nose to bleed. Then he has to lie flat with cotton wool in his nostrils. He sneezes once again and blows out the cotton wool, which aggravates the bleeding.. The G.P. thinks it must be an allergy to food so he is on Piriton allergy tablets which are not effective.

On October the panel classified this domain as High

CONTINENCE

High (the highest rating – it should be severe)

Continence Care is problematic and requires timely, urgent and skilled intervention.

Gerald is doubly incontinent and there are regular major crises, above and beyond what is normally understood as incontinence, when he loses complete faecal control, totally evacuates his bowels on the carpet and walks through the great volume of mess, often naked, with faeces coating his legs. Carpets have to be washed and he has to be showered.

I wash the sheets and the duvet. I wash the mattress and even the pillows

His clothes are so badly soiled that they often have to be thrown away (Accompanying letter from Host Carer)

I wash the chairs and the cushions. Swilling his clothes, even shoes and socks, and the cushions, in the kitchen sink my hands are in the filthy water full of faeces. I cannot put badly soiled articles straight into the washing machine without swilling them down and getting rid of most of the waste down the kitchen sink. It can take nearly 5 hours to clean him up, to clean the flat, the chairs and carpets and wash his clothes.

He loses complete control, and is not aware of what is happening and sometimes laughs. Cleaning him and his surroundings is a major exercise taking hours of work and distress. As his carer I am unable to control my feelings of desperation and distress when this happens.

He never remembers (even within a few seconds) what happened. Last time it took me five hours to clean the flat as well as him and swill his clothes for the washing machine.

Tests have been made by his G.P. to try to discover what triggers off these attacks but they are described by Dr Somerfield, his consultant, as 'cognitive.'

Previous October panel rated this as High

SKIN
High
High risk of skin breakdown which requires a minimum of daily monitoring or reassessment.

Gerald's skin has been described by the consultant at Torbay as 'paper thin.'

As a result of the skin on both his legs breaking down Gerald spent a week in Torbay hospital

He was diagnosed with Cellulitis, resulting in a general infection, a Urinary Tract Infection and 'Toxic Confusion'. He suffers from severe oedema in both legs.

He needs careful monitoring as he is very frail (**Torbay hospital notes 22/2/07 Note 5.**) '**...his skin is at risk of breakdown.**' Doctors verbal advice to me, his carer, was that he requires daily inspections and treatment twice a day, everyday, and that his skin is 'paper thin'. Therefore skin needs should be classified as **High.**

He requires regular daily inspections and treatment twice a day.

High rating – daily monitoring or reassessment

COMMUNICATION

Low

Needs assistance to communicate their needs. Special effort may be needed to ensure accurate interpretation of needs, or may need additional support either visually through touch or with hearing Carer may be able to anticipate needs due to familiarity with the individual.

Gerald does not communicate his needs.

In the last month, at home, he has become very withdrawn, and has ceased to converse.

His speech is hesitant

His vision is severely impaired. He is registered blind.

Skilled intervention/anticipation by Eleanor Graham, Host Carer, can pre-empt problems. In the past she managed to persuade him to talk about his life in the Navy, but recently that has ceased. His male carer is unable to persuade him to talk.

Low

BREATHING

Moderate

Episodes of breathlessness which do not respond to management but limit some daily activities.

Gerald has frequent attacks of hyperventilation and panting. ..Shortness of breath, Tachycardia and Chest pains – admitted to Simpson Ward, Torbay Hospital. (Feb 2005. Note 2ab)

His pulse rate increases during the attacks and he shows signs of distress for long periods when this happens

These attacks do not appear to be related to any particular cause or incident and occur so frequently that I have ceased to call for an ambulance. However they do interrupt daily life, such as taking him to church, or out in the car. His chest pains appear to be distressing and last for about an hour or more and his pulse rate rises.

Last time the ambulance was called they put him on oxygen and took him to hospital. He was in hospital for a week. Nowadays I do not wish to cause him anxiety by calling for an ambulance, or risk MRSA (as long as the problem begins to ease off within an hour)

Previous panel classified his condition as Moderate

DRUG THERAPY AND MEDICATION

Low

Requires supervision/administration of medication and has cognitive impairment requiring support to take medication, sometimes exhibits non-compliance with medication regime.

Gerald requires close supervision of his medication

Due to severe memory loss and blindness he requires prompting and assistance to take prescribed drugs. If he is not supervised he does not take his medication.

Because of his dysphagia he is unable to swallow his tablets and consequently he appears to chew them up which causes tooth decay and stomach problems. As a result he has lost six teeth which have fallen out leaving the roots exposed. His dentist does not wish to pursue further treatment as an anaesthetic would be too risky.

Low

ASC (Altered states of consciousness)

Low

This was classified as Low due to his suffering several TIAs

APPENDIX 2

The Case for Continuous Funding

It is contended that a person with Mr. Hill's condition should received NHS Continuing Care Funding. The Health Service has abandoned the care of my husband and passed that responsibility on to me. They have left me to sort out complex health problems arising from multiple care needs and I now require help which is beyond the scope of the Social Services remit as defined by section 49 of the Health and Social Care Act, and as a carer I am in need of urgent help as set out in the Carers Act 2000.

The case for the appeal is based on the following:

The *totality* of relevant needs, including other factors, such as blindness, have not been taken into account

The carers mental and physical health needs have not been adequately addressed.

The eligibility criteria for people with dementia and other sensory disabilities appear to lack as much sympathetic consideration on the aspects of their care as those with physical health needs.

Previous PCT assessments relied on inaccurate and inadequate information and therefore failed to take account of all the relevant facts. Their decisions conflicted, nor did they appear to have been given the actual copies of the papers that I had written for them, providing them with detailed information.

This resulted in my husband wrongly being refused NHS funding for care at home.

My husband's condition was diagnosed 6 years ago and now he has become severely disorientated and in need of full time care. It is unreasonable to believe that I should be expected to provide continuous care, especially at the age of 76 with my own medical problems as outlined in this document.

1) The totality of relevant needs.

The Appeal Court Judgement in the case of Pamela Coughlin (1999) and the remarks of the learned Judge in Grogan, advises that "You should address the totality of the relevant needs and answer the question as to whether the nature and degree of care, alone or *together with other factors,* means that the local authority cannot provide it in its totality, and therefore if it is to be provided, its provision falls on the NHS."

2.) The Eligibility Criteria

The Decision Support Tool of the Dept. of Health National Framework 2007 refers to cognitive impairment, mobility, continence, skin care management, behaviour, psychological and emotional needs and nutrition, which are rated very highly and are extremely relevant in my husband's case. However during his assessment for continuing care there has been no recognition of the difficulties of his increasing blindness which now severely compound most of his daily care needs.

It is to be stressed that Alzheimer's disease is a complex, debilitating physical and mental illness which in this case has been further compounded by heart problems, several TIAs, blindness and impaired kidney function as listed. Alzheimer's is by its nature an unstable condition whose progress is unpredictable and when assessing the total health needs of an individual, even though they are cared for at home, they are still eligible for Continuing NHS Health care. I would like to draw your attention to the findings of the Ombudsman in the Pointon Case –E22/02-03:

'In a situation such as this, with a patient whose mental and physical condition was inevitably going to deteriorate, it would seem short-sighted not to explore both the physical and psychological problems, with a view to the kind of support that would be needed in the near future.'

In addition, the four Priority categories of the Decision Support Tool (DST) reflect medical problems that would mainly apply to a patient cared for in a hospital or in a nursing home, <u>but the DST does not adequately assess the needs of a patient with dementia and physical needs cared for in his own home.</u> I maintain that the previous assessments made by the PCT were biased towards my husband's <u>physical</u> condition and were inappropriate for assessing the needs of people with dementia. They did not address my husband's needs, nor reflect the constant vigilance that is necessary to respond to the many unpredictable happenings in my husband's daily life.

Carer

It is an essential component of the assessment to identify the impact of the caring role on the carer in light of the carer's age, general health, status, interests and other commitments. No consideration has been given to my needs as a carer in accordance with the Carer's Act 2000, and I would further draw your attention to the findings of the Ombudsman in the Pointon Case –E22/02-03:

'The PCT may need to take into consideration the needs of carers, in accordance with the Carers Act 2000'

Gerald is totally dependent on me. Without me he could not survive. I am never able to relax my vigilance at all. Now, because of his deteriorating condition and behaviour, I require much more help.

I will be 77 years of age this year and suffer from a chronic kidney complaint (duplex kidney with reflux). As a child I was extremely ill with pylo-nephritis which went undiagnosed for a long period, following that frequent UTIs continued to damage both kidneys. Although this condition has been stabilised <u>I survive on little more than half a kidney</u>. I am on daily medication, Furadantin, for Urinary Tract infections and Atenolol for high blood pressure, and become physically tired and exhausted. As well as these problems I also suffer from severe pain and weakness in both wrists as a result of osteo-arthritis. In particular in my right wrist - so that I have difficulty dressing myself or my husband, using kitchen implements or carrying out normal day to day work. I have also been diagnosed with Type 2 Diabetes. In addition I have now been prescribed anti–depressant drugs as treatment for my own mental health problems – as a result of caring for my husband.

I note that when continuing care funding is granted, a carer is entitled to Respite care. As a carer I am expected to cope with this impossible situation without any respite whatsoever.

In a care home there is a team of carers, cooks and cleaners. In this home there is a team of one who is disabled by arthritis, impaired kidney function and depression.

I regularly fall deeply asleep several times a day and on 9th. May 2008 I crashed my car in a service station car park. On 16th May Dr Anderson at Parkhill Medical Practice diagnosed Mental Fatigue due to stress as my brain was unable to concentrate or function normally. She advised that my husband should spend a week or more in a care home as I needed a complete rest.

It should be borne in mind that a male carer comes in for half an hour in the evening and I am with my husband for the remaining twenty three and a half hours.

So in summary we think that Cognition and Continence should be rated Severe; Mobility, Psychological/Emotional and Skin needs should be High. Breathing needs should be classified as Moderate (limiting daily activities) We concur with the findings of the August 2008 panel that Behaviour and Nutrition should both be rated High and Communication should be classified as Low. However, taking into account the comments of the August 2008 Panel, Drug Therapies and Medication should be classified as Moderate due to Mr. Hill's non-compliance and non- concordance.

APPEAL

I would like to comment on the constant delays by the PCT to make arrangements for the hearings and the subsequent appeal.

20th. December 2006 Consideration by Health and Social Care Panel. Refusal

27th December 2006 I informed the Torbay PCT of my intention to appeal

31st January 2007 Reconsideration by Panel. Refusal

19th February 2007 I informed Torbay PCT of my intention to appeal once again

18th. July 2007 CPN assessment **(More than 5 months later)**

October 2007 Consideration by Panel. Refusal

21st. October 2007 Notification by me of appeal against the refusal of the PCT

Christmas 2007 I telephoned Torbay PCT to enquire about the date of the appeal. I was told that the PCT was hoping to get a panel together for the end of January. At the end of January I telephoned again and was informed that the Manager dealing with the appeal was on leave. I phoned again the following week and was informed that the Manager was 'off sick.'

In **February 2008** I wrote to Torbay PCT saying that I wished to cancel my appeal to the PCT and ask the Strategic Health Authority to consider the matter (see copy of my letter) as it was now 4 months since my application had been refused. I also wrote to the Chief Executive of the Strategic Health Authority enclosing a copy of that letter.

February 29th.2008 As there had been no response from either the PCT or the SHA I phoned the Strategic Health Authority today and was phoned back by Eileen Roberts of the SHA who informed me that I had to have my application to the PCT refused twice before I was able to appeal.

I pointed out that my application had been rejected on 20th December 2006, 31st. January 2007 and again in October 2007 and on each occasion I had been asked, in a letter from the PCT, if I wished to appeal. Within several days of receipt of those invitations I gave notice to the PCT that I did wish to appeal.

Eileen Roberts said that she would take up the matter with Torbay PCT and get back to me the following Monday. **These delays amounted to more than 9 months**.

19th.March 2008 **I telephoned Eileen Roberts (SHA), who apologised for not getting back to me, but explained that Torbay PCT has still been unable to carry out an Independent Review of my husband's condition. <u>Apparently the PCT has a backlog of cases which go back as far as 2004 and they have been instructed to clear these cases before dealing with other applications.</u>**

On 25th April 2008 Ann Redmayne, Health Commissioner, took up the matter with the PCT and in **May 2008** the PCT informed Claire Rowland, Care Manager, that they were still unable to set up an independent panel for the appeal and were contacting Cornwall to see whether they could assist in the matter.

On 23rd. May 2008 I received a letter from Alison Peters, Lead Nurse for the NHS Continuing Care Team setting out a plan of action.

On **28th. May 2008** Julie Cave from the Chadwell team phoned and made an appointment to re-assess Gerald's condition on **June 5th.**

The appeal was heard on **the 6th. August 2008** and was rejected several weeks later.

On **25th November 2008** I appealed to an independent panel set up by the South West Regional Health Authority. It is now **March 2009** and I have yet to hear the result.

I also cancelled the holiday I had booked in August 2008 to take Gerald for a week's holiday in Cornwall as I realised that I could no longer cope with him away from home, in a different setting – he has become so confused and regularly gets lost in his own home. The rows are getting worse and he is very aggressive. Also I asked Claire Rowland if she could arrange morning and evening visits from a carer to dress him in the morning and get him ready for bed in the evening. Hopefully if this could be arranged it might reduce the continual rows and noise he makes. However morning visits do not appear to be possible at present.

In conclusion I would end by pointing out that the Torbay PCT have let me down by ignoring the Core Values and Principles of the National Framework for NHS Continuing Health Care, and after 4 years, at the end of Dec 2007, re-assessed my needs as a carer (in compliance with the Carer's Act 2000) who provides daily and substantial care for Mr Hill. This assessment was due to my insistence.

You will be aware that once the updated assessment has been made, the local authority has a duty to take into account the results of that assessment when deciding what services to provide to the cared person. If the local authority believes that the provision of care for the cared person might be enhanced by the provision of services from another authority, then that authority must give due consideration to the request. Due consideration means that the authority to whom the request is made cannot fail to consider it, cannot dismiss it arbitrarily, or have a blanket ban on considering certain types of requests.

Finally I would ask that before reaching your decision you consider the findings of the Ombudsman in the Pointon Case which bears a close similarity to our own situation.

However I consider that it is vitally important to leave you with the knowledge that the Needs Portrayal Document presented to you by Torbay Primary Care Trust contains 94 matters all of which are dated. 58 of those dates are dated between one and two years ago - mostly in 2006 and quite a few in 2007 and should be viewed as completely out of date. The other 36 are dated during this year. My document is dated and is relevant to this year 2008. You will appreciate that a time lag of only a few weeks can considerably affect the condition and progress of Alzheimers disease.

Jane E. Hill 18/03/2009

Addendum 10/08/2009

Since my husband became a resident in Woodrow Retirement Home there have been several changes to his condition. Over the last four months Gerald's mental health has steadily deteriorated. He is more confused, probably due to the effect of the anaesthetic, the pain and discomfort and the fact that he has been moved from one hospital to another. The staff at Woodrow understand the effect of all this on him and do everything to make life as easy as possible. Nevertheless Alzheimers is a progressive illness and one must accept that his mental health will continue to deteriorate.

It is also believed that he may have a hair line crack in his femur which may account for his continuing pain and his Doctor has prescribed pain relief 4 times daily. It has also been agreed that a reclining chair should be provided for him. This should give him more relief.

Gerald has lost confidence in being able to walk again. He is still weak and has little enthusiasm or determination to persist in exercising. I have reached the conclusion that his attitude to exercise is 'Just leave me alone.' I can find no incentive to get him to make the effort. At his age of 88 he does not want to be bothered.

As for myself I find this distressing. I am suffering from stress, regularly falling asleep for many hours, also losing my balance and falling over injuring myself; smashing my car, breaking my hand and tearing a ligament in my leg. I do not seem to be able to come to terms with this situation. It distresses me to visit Gerald every day and see him steadily deteriorating. Yesterday we had afternoon tea and cakes in the garden. When I reminded him to eat his cake he pulled his handkerchief from his pocket and began to eat that. His incontinence problem is now much worse and more noticeable and I am relieved that he is not at home.

We have been married 56 years. My only relief is the knowledge that the staff at Woodrow Residential Home are looking after him very much better than I can, but I long to have the man that I married beside me once again.

Jane E. Hill 06/09/2009

The End